An All-Inclusive Heart Disease

Meal Diet

STEP-BY-STEP GUIDE TO

PREVENTING

and

TREATING

CARDIOVASCULAR

ISSUES,

hypertension + stroke
Coronary Artery Disease +
Heart Attack (Prior To 65
Years Of Age)

LUCIA DIAZ MATEO

An All-Inclusive Heart Disease Meal Diet

Step-By-Step Guide To
Preventing And Treating Cardiovascular Issues,

hypertension + stroke Coronary Artery Disease + Heart Attack (Prior To 65 Years Of Age)

By

Lucia Diaz Mateo

Copyright ©

CONTENTS

Chapter 1: Introduction

In the intricate tapestry of our lives, the role of nutrition is paramount, especially when it comes to the health of our hearts. Welcome to the exploration of an all-encompassing journey toward a heart disease meal diet – a step-by-step guide that unveils the intricate dance between what we consume and the well-being of our cardiovascular system. we embark on a profound understanding of how our dietary choices can significantly influence the prevention and treatment of heart-related issues, with a particular focus on hypertension, stroke, coronary artery disease (CAD), and heart attacks before the age of 65.

The Heart as a Vital Organ:

Our hearts, steadfastly beating from the moment we enter this world, serve as the epicenter of vitality. This magnificent organ pumps life-giving blood, carrying essential nutrients and oxygen to every nook and cranny of our bodies. However, this ceaseless rhythmic symphony can face challenges, often stemming from lifestyle choices, genetics, and environmental factors.

Linking Diet and Cardiovascular Health:

The intricate relationship between diet and heart health is not a new revelation, yet its significance is often underestimated. What we consume directly influences the health of our arteries, blood pressure, and overall cardiovascular function. Recognizing this connection becomes the first crucial step in taking charge of our heart's destiny.

Purpose of this Guide:

The primary aim of this comprehensive guide is to empower you with the knowledge and tools needed to make informed dietary choices that will contribute to the prevention and treatment of cardiovascular issues. By delving into the intricacies of nutrition, we aim to provide you with a roadmap to cultivate a heart-healthy lifestyle that extends beyond the immediate concerns, fostering longevity and vitality.

Holistic Approach:

This guide adopts a holistic approach to heart health. It's not just about what you eat; it's about understanding the synergy between different elements of your lifestyle. From mindful eating practices to the incorporation of heart-boosting superfoods, we will navigate the multifaceted landscape of cardiovascular well-being.

Acknowledging the Challenge:

Embarking on a journey to transform dietary habits can be daunting, but it is an investment in your future self. We acknowledge the challenges you may face and are here to guide you, step by step, through the process. Whether you are seeking preventive measures or aiming to manage existing conditions, this guide is designed to be your companion, providing insights, practical tips, and a wealth of information to support your endeavor.

The Road Ahead:

As we unfold the layers of a heart-healthy meal diet, each subsequent chapter will delve into specific aspects of nutrition, addressing hypertension, stroke, CAD, heart attacks, and the unique considerations for individuals under 65 years of age. The journey is not only about understanding the science behind the food we eat but also about fostering a mindful and sustainable approach to nourishing our bodies.

Chapter 2: Foundation of a Heart-Healthy Diet

A robust foundation is crucial when embarking on a journey to maintain or improve heart health through dietary choices. The foundation of a heart-healthy diet lies in understanding the essential nutrients that play a pivotal role in cardiovascular well-being. By grasping the significance of these nutrients and incorporating them into our daily meals, we lay the groundwork for a preventive and supportive approach to heart health.

Understanding Macronutrients:

The first pillar of our foundation is macronutrients – carbohydrates, proteins, and fats. Balancing these macronutrients is key to promoting heart health. Carbohydrates, sourced from whole grains, fruits, and vegetables, provide energy and essential fiber. Fiber, in particular, aids in managing cholesterol levels and promoting a healthy digestive system.

Proteins, derived from lean sources like poultry, fish, legumes, and nuts, contribute to muscle health and repair. Including a variety of protein sources ensures a well-rounded intake of essential amino acids, crucial for overall bodily functions.

Fats, often misunderstood, include both healthy and unhealthy varieties. Emphasizing unsaturated fats found in olive oil, avocados, and fatty fish supports cardiovascular health. These fats assist in reducing bad cholesterol levels while promoting the presence of good cholesterol.

The Power of Micronutrients:

Micronutrients, including vitamins and minerals, form the second pillar of our foundation. These play a crucial role in supporting various physiological functions necessary for heart health. Key vitamins such as Vitamin C, found in citrus fruits, and Vitamin E, present in nuts and seeds, act as antioxidants, combating free radicals that contribute to heart disease.

Minerals like potassium, magnesium, and calcium contribute to maintaining proper blood pressure and heart rhythm. Foods such as bananas, leafy greens, and dairy products are rich sources of these essential minerals.

Antioxidants and Heart Health:

The third pillar revolves around antioxidants, powerful compounds that neutralize oxidative stress in the body. Berries, dark chocolate, and colorful vegetables are abundant in antioxidants, protecting the heart from damage caused by free radicals. Including a diverse array of antioxidant-rich foods adds a layer of defense against inflammation and arterial damage.

Omega-3 Fatty Acids:

Omega-3 fatty acids, predominantly found in fatty fish like salmon and mackerel, walnuts, and flaxseeds, constitute the fourth pillar. These essential fatty acids have been linked to a lower risk of heart disease by reducing inflammation, improving cholesterol levels, and supporting overall heart function.

Balancing Sodium and Potassium:

The fifth and final pillar addresses the delicate balance between sodium and potassium. Excessive sodium intake, often linked to processed foods, can elevate blood pressure and strain the heart. On the other hand, potassium, prevalent in bananas, sweet potatoes, and leafy greens, helps counteract the adverse effects of sodium, maintaining a healthy blood pressure range.

In essence, the foundation of a heart-healthy diet rests upon a thoughtful combination of macronutrients, micronutrients, antioxidants, omega-3 fatty acids, and a mindful balance between sodium and potassium. Armed with this understanding, individuals can make informed choices when crafting meals that not only satisfy taste buds but also nourish and protect the heart.

Chapter 3: Assessing Your Current Diet - Identifying Red Flags and Unhealthy Habits

Understanding the current state of your dietary habits is a crucial step in the journey towards a heart-healthy lifestyle. This aims to guide you through a comprehensive assessment, helping you identify potential red flags and unhealthy patterns that may contribute to cardiovascular issues.

I. Self-Reflection on Eating Patterns

Begin by reflecting on your typical eating patterns. Consider your meal timings, portion sizes, and frequency of snacks. Are you often eating on-the-go, neglecting balanced meals? Reflecting on these aspects can provide valuable insights into areas that may need improvement.

II. Food Diary Analysis

Keeping a food diary is a powerful tool for self-awareness. Record everything you consume over a week, including beverages and snacks. Analyze the entries to identify patterns – are there excessive amounts of processed foods, sugary drinks, or high-sodium items? This detailed record will serve as a foundation for making informed adjustments to your diet.

III. Nutrient Intake Evaluation

Assess the balance of macronutrients (carbohydrates, proteins, and fats) in your diet. Are you consuming an excess of unhealthy fats, such as saturated and trans fats? Is there a lack of essential nutrients like fiber, vitamins, and minerals? Understanding your nutrient intake helps pinpoint areas where modifications can enhance heart health.

IV. Sodium Awareness

Examine your sodium intake, a critical factor in hypertension and overall heart health. Processed foods and restaurant meals often contain hidden sodium. Identifying sources of high sodium in your diet can help you make conscious choices to reduce intake and protect your cardiovascular system.

V. Sugar and Sweetener Evaluation

Assess your sugar consumption, including both added sugars and natural sugars. High sugar intake is linked to various heart-related issues. Identify sources of added sugars in your diet, such as sugary beverages, snacks, and desserts.

Exploring alternatives and reducing reliance on

excessive sweeteners can significantly benefit your

heart.

VI. Alcohol Consumption Analysis

Evaluate your alcohol consumption patterns. While moderate alcohol intake may have cardiovascular benefits, excessive or frequent drinking can contribute to heart issues. Understanding your alcohol habits allows you to make informed decisions regarding moderation for heart health.

VII. Fruits and Vegetables Assessment

Analyze your fruit and vegetable intake. These nutrient-rich foods play a vital role in heart health. Identify opportunities to increase the variety and quantity of colorful, fresh produce in your meals, ensuring a rich supply of antioxidants and essential nutrients.

VIII. Hydration Habits

Examine your hydration habits. Water is fundamental to overall health, including heart function. Assess whether you're meeting daily hydration needs and consider reducing reliance on sugary drinks or excessive caffeinated beverages.

IX. Meal Timing and Frequency

Evaluate your meal timing and frequency. Irregular eating patterns or skipping meals can impact blood sugar levels and metabolism, potentially affecting heart health. Establishing consistent and balanced meal routines contributes to a stable and nourished cardiovascular system.

X. Emotional and Stress-Related Eating

Reflect on emotional and stress-related eating. Understand if your diet is influenced by emotions or stress, leading to unhealthy choices. Developing mindfulness around emotional eating provides a foundation for cultivating healthier coping mechanisms.

By thoroughly assessing your current diet through these key dimensions, you gain valuable insights into areas that require attention and modification. This self-awareness lays the groundwork for the subsequent chapters, where we'll delve into specific strategies and dietary adjustments to foster a heart-healthy lifestyle. Remember, small changes can lead to significant improvements in your cardiovascular well-being.

Chapter 4: Key Elements of a Preventive Meal Plan

Maintaining heart health involves more than just avoiding certain foods; it requires a proactive approach centered around a well-crafted preventive meal plan. the key elements that constitute an effective diet for preventing cardiovascular issues such as hypertension, stroke, coronary artery disease, and heart attacks before the age of 65.

Understanding Nutritional Foundations

Before we dive into specific dietary recommendations, it's crucial to grasp the nutritional foundations that support heart health. Essential nutrients play a pivotal role in maintaining optimal cardiovascular function. These include omega-3 fatty acids, antioxidants, fiber, vitamins (especially B-complex and D), and minerals like potassium and magnesium.

Balancing Macronutrients

One of the cornerstones of a heart-healthy diet is achieving a balance between macronutrients. While each macronutrient plays a role, an emphasis on the quality of fats is particularly important. Replace saturated and trans fats with heart-healthy unsaturated fats, found in olive oil, avocados, and nuts. Additionally, focus on lean sources of protein, such as fish, poultry, and legumes, and choose whole grains over refined carbohydrates for a stable source of energy.

Incorporating Antioxidants

Antioxidants are potent compounds that counteract oxidative stress in the body. Including a variety of fruits and vegetables in your diet ensures a diverse range of antioxidants, protecting your heart from damage caused by free radicals. Berries, leafy greens, tomatoes, and citrus fruits are rich sources of these protective compounds.

Omega-3 Fatty Acids for Heart Health

Omega-3 fatty acids, particularly eicosapentaenoic acid (EPA) and docosahexaenoic acid (DHA), have been extensively studied for their cardiovascular benefits. These fatty acids, found in fatty fish like salmon, mackerel, and walnuts, help reduce inflammation, lower blood triglycerides, and support overall heart function. Consider incorporating fish into your diet at least twice a week for a reliable source of omega-3s.

Strategic Use of Fiber

Dietary fiber is a multifaceted ally in heart health. It helps control cholesterol levels, regulates blood sugar, and promotes a healthy gut microbiome. Opt for whole grains, legumes, fruits, and vegetables to increase your fiber intake. Additionally, consuming soluble fiber, found in oats, barley, and fruits, can contribute to lowering LDL cholesterol levels.

Hydration and Heart Function

Adequate hydration is often overlooked but is fundamental for maintaining cardiovascular health. Water supports blood volume and helps transport nutrients and oxygen to cells. Dehydration can strain the heart and lead to elevated blood pressure. Aim for at least 8 glasses of water a day, adjusting based on factors like climate and physical activity.

Limiting Added Sugars and Refined Carbohydrates

Excessive consumption of added sugars and refined carbohydrates has been linked to an increased risk of heart disease. These foods contribute to inflammation, insulin resistance, and weight gain. Be mindful of sugary beverages, candies, and processed snacks, and opt for whole, unprocessed foods to provide sustained energy without the negative cardiovascular impact.

Minimizing Sodium Intake

Excessive sodium intake is a major contributor to hypertension. Processed and restaurant-prepared foods often contain high levels of hidden salt. Reading food labels, cooking at home, and flavoring meals with herbs and spices instead of salt can help manage sodium intake. Aim to keep daily sodium consumption within the recommended guidelines for heart health.

Individualizing the Preventive Meal Plan

While these general guidelines provide a solid foundation, it's essential to recognize that individual nutritional needs vary. Factors such as age, gender, activity level, and existing health conditions influence dietary requirements. Consulting with a healthcare professional or a registered dietitian can help tailor a preventive meal plan to your specific needs, ensuring a more personalized and effective approach to heart health.

Chapter 5: Navigating Hypertension - Dietary Strategies to Manage and Lower Blood Pressure

Hypertension, commonly known as high blood pressure, is a prevalent cardiovascular condition that requires careful attention to dietary choices.

relationship between food and blood pressure, offering a comprehensive guide to help you navigate hypertension effectively.

Understanding Hypertension:

Hypertension is a condition where the force of blood against the walls of the arteries is consistently too high. It is often referred to as the "silent killer" because it may not present noticeable symptoms, yet it significantly increases the risk of heart disease, stroke, and other health issues.

Dietary Impact on Blood Pressure:

Your dietary choices play a crucial role in managing blood pressure. Certain nutrients can either contribute to or alleviate hypertension. Let's explore the key dietary strategies to help you maintain a healthy blood pressure level.

1. Mindful Sodium Consumption:

Sodium, a component of salt, is a major contributor to elevated blood pressure. Processed foods, canned goods, and restaurant meals often contain high levels of sodium. In this section,

2. Potassium-Rich Foods:

Potassium counteracts the effects of sodium, helping to regulate blood pressure. The potassium-rich foods like bananas, oranges, and leafy greens, and you can provide creative ways to incorporate them into your daily meals.

3. Magnesium and Calcium Balance:

The delicate balance between magnesium and calcium is crucial for maintaining healthy blood pressure.

4. Fiber and Whole Grains:

A diet high in fiber and whole grains has been associated with lower blood pressure levels.

5. Healthy Fats and Omega-3s:

Certain fats, like those found in avocados, nuts, and fatty fish, have been linked to lower blood pressure.

6. Limiting Alcohol Intake:

Excessive alcohol consumption can contribute to hypertension.

7. DASH Diet Principles:

The Dietary Approaches to Stop Hypertension (DASH) diet is a well-researched approach to lowering blood pressure through dietary changes. We'll break down the key principles of the DASH diet and offer practical tips for integrating them into your daily life.

8. Fluid Balance and Hydration:

Adequate hydration is essential for overall health, including maintaining blood pressure.

Chapter 6: Decoding Stroke Prevention

Stroke, often referred to as a "brain attack," is a severe medical condition that occurs when blood flow to the brain is disrupted. The consequences can be devastating, making stroke prevention a critical aspect of maintaining overall cardiovascular health.

We will explore the intricate relationship between diet and stroke prevention, delving into the foods that support brain health and reduce the risk of this life-altering event.

Understanding Stroke Risk Factors:

Before delving into dietary strategies, it's crucial to understand the risk factors associated with strokes. Hypertension, diabetes, high cholesterol levels, and smoking are common contributors to stroke risk. Additionally, age, family history, and certain medical conditions can increase susceptibility. Armed with this knowledge, we can tailor our dietary approach to address these risk factors.

The Power of Antioxidant-Rich Foods:

Antioxidants play a pivotal role in protecting the body from oxidative stress, a factor implicated in stroke development. Including a variety of colorful fruits and vegetables in your diet ensures a diverse range of antioxidants. Berries, rich in anthocyanins, have shown particular promise in supporting brain health. Dark leafy greens, nuts, and seeds are also excellent sources of antioxidants that contribute to overall vascular well-being.

Omega-3 Fatty Acids: Guardians of Brain Health:

Omega-3 fatty acids, especially EPA and DHA found in fatty fish like salmon and mackerel, have been extensively studied for their neuroprotective properties. These essential fatty acids contribute to the maintenance of healthy blood vessels, reducing the risk of clot formation and promoting optimal blood flow to the brain. For those not inclined towards fish, flaxseeds, chia seeds, and walnuts are plant-based alternatives rich in alpha-linolenic acid (ALA), a precursor to EPA and DHA.

Balancing Sodium Intake:

Excessive sodium intake can contribute to hypertension, a significant stroke risk factor. Reducing salt in the diet involves not only limiting the use of the salt shaker but also being mindful of hidden sodium in processed foods. Embracing fresh, whole foods and cooking at home allows for better control over sodium intake. Herbs and spices can be delightful alternatives to enhance flavor without relying on excessive salt.

Emphasizing Potassium-Rich Foods:

Potassium plays a crucial role in counteracting the negative effects of sodium on blood pressure. Incorporating potassium-rich foods, such as bananas, oranges, spinach, and sweet potatoes, can help maintain a healthy balance. These foods not only contribute to blood pressure regulation but also support overall cardiovascular health.

The Mediterranean Diet and Stroke Prevention:

Numerous studies have highlighted the benefits of the Mediterranean diet in reducing stroke risk. This diet emphasizes fruits, vegetables, whole grains, nuts, seeds, and olive oil while limiting red meat and processed foods. The abundance of antioxidants, omega-3 fatty acids, and other essential nutrients in this diet contributes to its stroke-preventive qualities.

Limiting Alcohol Consumption:

While moderate alcohol consumption has been associated with certain cardiovascular benefits, excessive alcohol intake can elevate blood pressure and increase the risk of stroke. If you choose to consume alcohol, it's essential to do so in moderation. For those who don't drink, there's no need to start, as the risks may outweigh the potential benefits.

The Role of Fiber in Stroke Prevention:

Dietary fiber offers a myriad of benefits, and stroke prevention is no exception. Whole grains, legumes, fruits, and vegetables are excellent sources of fiber that contribute to heart health. Fiber helps regulate blood pressure, control cholesterol levels, and support overall vascular function. Additionally, it promotes a healthy gut microbiome, which has emerging links to cardiovascular well-being.

Hydration and Its Impact on Stroke Risk:

Staying adequately hydrated is fundamental to overall health, and it also plays a role in stroke prevention. Dehydration can lead to thicker blood, making clot formation more likely. Ensuring sufficient water intake contributes to optimal blood viscosity and circulation. Herbal teas and infused water can add variety while keeping hydration levels in check.

Customizing Your Stroke-Prevention Diet:

It's essential to recognize that there's no one-size-fits-all approach to stroke prevention through diet. Individual dietary needs vary based on factors such as age, health status, and personal preferences. Consulting with a healthcare professional or a registered dietitian can help tailor a plan that aligns with your specific requirements and addresses potential risk factors.

Chapter 7: Combatting Coronary Artery Disease (CAD) - Tailoring Your Diet to Protect Heart Arteries

Coronary Artery Disease (CAD) poses a significant threat to heart health, often arising from the gradual buildup of plaque in the coronary arteries. This chapter delves into the intricacies of CAD and how a well-crafted diet can be a powerful ally in preventing and managing this condition.

Understanding CAD:

Coronary Artery Disease occurs when the blood vessels supplying the heart muscle with oxygen and nutrients (coronary arteries) become narrowed or blocked by a buildup of cholesterol and other substances, forming plaque. This restricts blood flow to the heart, leading to various complications, including angina and heart attacks.

The Role of Diet in CAD:

Diet plays a pivotal role in the development and progression of CAD. Certain dietary choices can contribute to elevated cholesterol levels, hypertension, and inflammation, all of which are major risk factors for CAD. On the flip side, a heart-healthy diet can help manage these risk factors and even reverse the damage to some extent.

Emphasizing Heart-Protective Foods:

In the battle against CAD, it's crucial to incorporate foods that actively promote heart health. Omega-3 fatty acids found in fatty fish like salmon and mackerel, as well as walnuts and flaxseeds, have been shown to reduce inflammation and lower the risk of CAD. Fiber-rich foods such as whole grains, fruits, and vegetables contribute to better cholesterol levels and overall cardiovascular health.

Balancing Fats:

Not all fats are created equal, and understanding this distinction is key to combating CAD. While saturated and trans fats can contribute to elevated cholesterol, unsaturated fats – found in olive oil, avocados, and nuts – can have a protective effect. Striking a balance and making thoughtful fat choices are crucial components of a CAD-focused diet.

Limiting Processed Foods and Added Sugars:

Processed foods often contain unhealthy trans fats, excess sodium, and added sugars, all of which can exacerbate CAD risk factors. By reducing the intake of processed and sugary foods, individuals can positively impact their cholesterol levels, blood pressure, and overall heart health.

Incorporating Antioxidants:

Antioxidants play a vital role in reducing oxidative stress and inflammation, both of which are linked to CAD. Berries, dark chocolate, and colorful fruits and vegetables are rich sources of antioxidants that can be easily incorporated into a heart-protective diet.

The Mediterranean Diet Approach:

The Mediterranean diet has gained acclaim for its heart-healthy benefits, with an emphasis on fruits, vegetables, whole grains, lean proteins, and olive oil. Studies have shown that adopting a Mediterranean-style eating pattern can significantly reduce the risk of CAD and improve overall cardiovascular health.

Customizing the Diet to Individual Needs:

CAD is a complex condition influenced by various factors, including genetics and lifestyle. Therefore, it's essential to tailor the diet to individual needs. Consulting with a healthcare professional or a registered dietitian can help create a personalized plan that addresses specific risk factors and dietary requirements.

The Impact of Lifestyle Choices:

While diet is a powerful tool in CAD prevention, it works in conjunction with other lifestyle choices.

Quitting smoking, managing stress through techniques like meditation or yoga, and engaging in regular physical activity are integral components of a comprehensive approach to heart health.

Chapter 8: Understanding Heart Attack Risks - Dietary Measures to Reduce Vulnerability

A heart attack is a frightening and life-altering event that often results from a culmination of lifestyle factors, genetics, and underlying health conditions.

1. Unveiling Heart Attack Triggers

Heart attacks are often triggered by atherosclerosis, the buildup of plaque in the coronary arteries. Understanding this process is crucial to developing an effective preventive diet. Excessive consumption of saturated and trans fats, along with high levels of cholesterol, contributes to the development of arterial plaque. Therefore, a dietary focus on reducing these elements becomes paramount.

2. Cholesterol Management Through Diet

Dietary cholesterol plays a pivotal role in heart health. While the body requires cholesterol for various functions, excessive levels can lead to arterial blockages. Incorporating foods rich in soluble fiber, such as oats, beans, and fruits, can help lower cholesterol levels. Additionally, replacing saturated fats with healthy fats like those found in avocados, nuts, and olive oil can have a positive

impact.

3. Omega-3 Fatty Acids for Cardiovascular Defense

Omega-3 fatty acids, found in fatty fish like salmon, mackerel, and flaxseeds, have been proven to reduce the risk of heart attacks. These essential fats have anti-inflammatory properties, helping to maintain the elasticity of blood vessels and lower the likelihood of clot formation. Including omega-3-rich foods in your regular diet is a proactive step towards protecting your heart.

4. Antioxidants and Their Shielding Effect

Free radicals in the body can contribute to oxidative stress, promoting inflammation and damage to blood vessels. Antioxidants, abundant in fruits, vegetables, and nuts, neutralize these free radicals. By embracing a diet rich in colorful produce, you provide your body with the tools to combat oxidative stress and enhance cardiovascular resilience.

5. The Impact of Salt on Heart Health

Excessive salt intake has been linked to hypertension, a significant risk factor for heart attacks. Monitoring and reducing salt consumption is a critical aspect of a heart-healthy diet. Choosing fresh, whole foods over processed and packaged options helps control sodium intake. Herbs and spices can be excellent alternatives for flavoring meals without relying on excessive salt.

6. Balancing Blood Sugar Levels

Maintaining stable blood sugar levels is essential for heart health. Diets high in refined sugars and carbohydrates can lead to insulin resistance and an increased risk of heart disease. Opting for complex carbohydrates, such as whole grains, and incorporating foods that regulate blood sugar, like cinnamon and chromium-rich vegetables, supports overall cardiovascular well-being.

7. Moderating Alcohol Intake

While moderate alcohol consumption has been associated with certain heart benefits, excessive drinking can elevate the risk of heart attacks. It's crucial to understand and adhere to recommended limits. If you choose to consume alcohol, doing so responsibly and being mindful of its impact on your health is vital.

8. The Role of Nutrient-Rich Foods

Focusing on nutrient-dense foods ensures that your body receives essential vitamins and minerals crucial for heart health. Magnesium, potassium, and calcium are particularly important. Green leafy vegetables, nuts, seeds, and dairy products are excellent sources of these nutrients. A well-balanced and diverse diet contributes to overall cardiovascular resilience.

9. Hydration as a Heart Health Strategy

Adequate hydration is often overlooked but plays a significant role in heart health. Water helps maintain blood volume, preventing the blood from becoming too thick and reducing the workload on the heart. Staying well-hydrated supports the overall function of the cardiovascular system.

10. Customizing Dietary Strategies Based on Individual Risk Factors

It's essential to recognize that individuals have varying risk factors for heart attacks. Factors such as family history, age, and existing health conditions contribute to the overall risk profile. Consulting with a healthcare professional or a registered dietitian can provide personalized guidance on tailoring your diet to address specific risk factors.

Chapter 9: Age-Specific Nutrition Guidelines

As we journey through life, our nutritional needs evolve, and a tailored approach to diet becomes increasingly crucial. age-specific nutrition guidelines, recognizing the distinct requirements for optimal heart health at different life stages.

Early Years (0-5): Laying the Foundation

In the early years of life, nutrition plays a fundamental role in the development of a healthy heart. Breastfeeding provides essential nutrients and fosters a strong immune system. As solid foods are introduced, a focus on nutrient-dense options like fruits, vegetables, and whole grains establishes a foundation for lifelong heart health.

Childhood (6-12): Cultivating Healthy Habits

During childhood, the emphasis shifts to cultivating healthy eating habits. Encouraging a balanced diet with adequate fruits, vegetables, lean proteins, and whole grains contributes to the maintenance of a healthy weight and sets the stage for a heart-conscious adolescence.

Adolescence (13-18): Navigating Growth Spurts

The adolescent years bring rapid growth and development, demanding increased energy and nutrient intake. It's vital to balance the higher caloric needs with nutrient-rich foods, steering away from excessive processed sugars and unhealthy fats. Educating teenagers about mindful eating fosters a lifelong appreciation for nutrition.

Early Adulthood (19-30): Building a Solid Base

As individuals transition into early adulthood, establishing a solid nutritional base becomes paramount. Adequate intake of calcium, vitamin D, and omega-3 fatty acids supports bone health and cardiovascular function. This stage is also an opportune time to foster heart-healthy cooking skills and mindful eating practices that can be carried into later years.

Adulthood (31-50): Maintaining Balance

Adulthood often comes with increased responsibilities and potential stressors. Maintaining a balanced diet rich in antioxidants, fiber, and heart-healthy fats becomes essential. Regular exercise complements nutritional efforts, contributing to weight management and overall cardiovascular well-being.

Pre-Retirement (51-64): Anticipating Changes

Approaching the pre-retirement years, individuals may start experiencing hormonal shifts and metabolic changes. It becomes crucial to monitor cholesterol levels and blood pressure, adjusting the diet to accommodate these shifts. A focus on heart-boosting nutrients, such as potassium and magnesium, aids in maintaining optimal cardiovascular function.

Chapter 10: Mindful Eating Practices

In the quest for a heart-healthy lifestyle, the significance of mindful eating cannot be overstated.

relationship between emotional well-being and heart health, emphasizing the need for a mindful approach to nutrition.

Mindful eating is more than just a trend; it's a transformative practice that reconnects individuals with the present moment and fosters a deeper appreciation for the food on their plates.

As we explore the links between mindfulness and heart health, it's essential to understand that our mental state can significantly impact our dietary choices and, consequently, our cardiovascular well-being.

Mindful Awareness and Emotional Eating

One of the primary aspects of mindful eating is cultivating awareness. Many individuals find themselves caught in the cycle of emotional eating, using food as a coping mechanism for stress, anxiety, or boredom.

Mindful awareness encourages a pause before reaching for that snack, allowing individuals to assess their emotional state and choose a healthier response.

By developing a heightened awareness of emotional triggers, individuals can break free from the automatic patterns of emotional eating. This not only promotes better mental health but also contributes to a more heart-healthy lifestyle.

The Mind-Heart Connection

Research has shown a strong connection between mental health and heart health. Chronic stress, for example, can lead to the release of stress hormones like cortisol, which, over time, may contribute to inflammation and cardiovascular issues. Mindful eating acts as a powerful tool to manage stress, providing a way to engage with food in a manner that promotes relaxation and balance.

Moreover, mindful eating supports a positive mindset, fostering gratitude for the nourishment provided by each meal. This positive outlook can have a cascading effect on overall well-being, influencing factors like blood pressure and heart rate.

Practical Tips for Mindful Eating

1. Slow Down and savor: Eating slowly allows your body to recognize signals of fullness, preventing overeating. Take the time to savor the flavors, textures, and aromas of your food.

2. Eliminate distractions:

Turn off the TV, put away your phone, and create a peaceful environment for your meals. Distractions can lead to mindless eating and a disconnect from the experience of nourishing your body.

3. Listen to your body:

Pay attention to hunger and fullness cues. Eat when you're hungry, and stop when you're satisfied. This simple practice can prevent unnecessary calorie consumption and promote a healthier weight.

4. Engage your senses: Use all your senses to fully experience your meal. Notice the colors, smells, and textures of the food. This sensory engagement enhances the overall eating experience.

5. Practice gratitude: Before you begin your meal, take a moment to express gratitude for the nourishment in front of you. This mental shift can enhance the positive impact of your food on both your body and mind.

Mindful Eating and Dietary Choices

Incorporating mindfulness into your eating habits can influence the types of foods you choose. A mindful approach encourages a focus on nutrient-dense, whole foods that support heart health. When you are attuned to your body's needs and signals, you are more likely to make choices that align with long-term well-being.

Chapter 11: Balancing Macronutrients for Heart Health

Achieving a heart-healthy lifestyle involves more than just choosing the right foods; it requires a nuanced understanding of macronutrients and how they impact cardiovascular well-being. In this chapter, we will delve into the intricate dance between carbohydrates, proteins, and fats, exploring how the right balance can play a pivotal role in maintaining optimal heart health.

Understanding Macronutrients: The Building Blocks of Nutrition

Macronutrients are the essential components of our diet that provide the energy necessary for our body's functions. Carbohydrates, proteins, and fats each serve distinct roles, and their proportions in our diet can significantly influence heart health.

Carbohydrates: The Energy Source

Carbohydrates are our body's primary source of energy. However, not all carbs are created equal. Simple carbohydrates, found in sugary snacks and refined grains, can lead to rapid spikes in blood sugar, potentially stressing the cardiovascular system. On the other hand, complex carbohydrates, like those in whole grains and vegetables, provide sustained energy and contribute to overall heart health.

Proteins: The Building Blocks

Proteins are crucial for the repair and maintenance of tissues, including the heart muscle. Lean sources of protein, such as poultry, fish, legumes, and nuts, should be prioritized. These choices not only support heart health but also help maintain a healthy weight, reducing the risk of cardiovascular issues.

Fats: Choosing the Right Ones

Dietary fats are often misunderstood, but they play a vital role in heart health. Healthy fats, such as those found in avocados, olive oil, and fatty fish, can actually protect against cardiovascular diseases. On the other hand, trans fats and saturated fats, commonly found in processed and fried foods, can elevate cholesterol levels and increase the risk of heart problems.

The Heart-Healthy Balance: Proportions Matter

Balancing macronutrients is not a one-size-fits-all endeavor. The optimal proportions depend on various factors, including age, activity level, and individual health goals. However, general guidelines exist to help create a heart-healthy diet.

Emphasizing Whole Foods

Whole foods, such as fruits, vegetables, whole grains, and lean proteins, should form the foundation of a heart-healthy diet. These foods provide a rich array of nutrients while minimizing the intake of processed and refined products that can contribute to heart issues.

Moderating Carbohydrate Intake

While carbohydrates are essential, excessive consumption, especially of refined sugars and grains, can lead to weight gain and insulin resistance. Opt for complex carbohydrates and monitor portion sizes to maintain stable blood sugar levels.

Prioritizing Lean Proteins

Choose lean sources of protein to support muscle health without introducing excess saturated fats. Fish, poultry, legumes, and plant-based protein sources can be excellent choices.

Incorporating Healthy Fats

Healthy fats, such as monounsaturated and polyunsaturated fats, play a crucial role in cardiovascular health. Avocados, nuts, seeds, and olive oil are rich sources of these heart-friendly fats.

Fine-Tuning for Your Heart: Personalized Approaches

While general guidelines provide a solid foundation, individualization is key when it comes to balancing macronutrients for heart health.

Factors like pre-existing health conditions, dietary preferences, and lifestyle choices should all be considered in crafting a personalized approach.

Addressing Special Dietary Needs

Individuals with specific health conditions, such as diabetes or metabolic disorders, may require tailored macronutrient ratios. Consulting with a healthcare professional or a registered dietitian can help create a personalized plan that aligns with both nutritional needs and heart health goals.

Adapting to Physical Activity Levels

Active individuals may require a different macronutrient balance than those with a sedentary lifestyle. Athletes, for example, might benefit from a higher proportion of carbohydrates to fuel their energy-intensive activities.

Practical Tips for Balancing Macronutrients in Your Diet

1. Meal Planning

Prepare well-balanced meals ahead of time, ensuring a mix of carbohydrates, proteins, and fats in each serving.

2. Portion Control

Be mindful of portion sizes to prevent overconsumption of any particular macronutrient.

3. Diverse Protein Sources

Include a variety of protein sources in your diet to ensure a broad spectrum of essential amino acids.

4. Healthy Cooking Methods

Opt for cooking methods that preserve the nutritional value of foods, such as grilling, baking, or steaming.

5. Read Labels

Stay informed about the nutritional content of packaged foods, especially paying attention to hidden sugars and unhealthy fats.

Chapter 12: Heart-Boosting Superfoods

In the quest for a heart-healthy diet, the role of superfoods cannot be overstated. These nutrient-packed powerhouses go beyond mere sustenance; they actively contribute to cardiovascular well-being. Incorporating a variety of these superfoods into your daily meals can be a delicious and effective strategy for maintaining heart health.

1. Berries: The Antioxidant Heroes

Berries, such as blueberries, strawberries, and raspberries, are rich in antioxidants known as polyphenols. These compounds have been linked to reducing oxidative stress and inflammation, two factors implicated in heart disease. Including a handful of berries in your breakfast or as a snack can be a flavorful way to boost heart protection.

2. Fatty Fish: Omega-3 Rich Delicacies

Salmon, mackerel, and trout are not just delectable choices; they are also abundant in omega-3 fatty acids. These essential fats are renowned for their heart-protective benefits, including lowering blood pressure and reducing the risk of heart rhythm abnormalities. Aim for at least two servings of fatty fish per week to harness the cardiovascular advantages.

3. Nuts and Seeds: Crunchy Nutrient Powerhouses

Almonds, walnuts, flaxseeds, and chia seeds are packed with heart-healthy nutrients. These include omega-3 fatty acids, fiber, and antioxidants. Snacking on a handful of nuts or incorporating seeds into your meals provides a satisfying crunch while promoting heart wellness.

4. Dark Leafy Greens: Nutrient-Rich Greens

Spinach, kale, and Swiss chard are among the dark leafy greens that offer a plethora of vitamins, minerals, and antioxidants. These greens are particularly rich in potassium, a mineral linked to blood pressure regulation. Whether in salads, smoothies, or sautés, dark leafy greens are versatile additions to a heart-healthy diet.

5. Oats: Soluble Fiber for Cholesterol Management

Oats contain beta-glucans, a type of soluble fiber known for its cholesterol-lowering properties. Consuming oats regularly can contribute to maintaining healthy cholesterol levels, a crucial factor in preventing coronary artery disease. Start your day with a bowl of oatmeal topped with berries for a heart-boosting combination.

6. Avocado: Creamy Goodness with Healthy Fats

Avocado is a unique fruit rich in monounsaturated fats, which have been associated with improved heart health. These healthy fats help lower bad cholesterol levels while increasing good cholesterol. Spread avocado on whole-grain toast or add slices to salads for a creamy and heart-friendly touch.

7. Tomatoes: Lycopene for Cardiovascular Support

Tomatoes contain lycopene, a powerful antioxidant with potential heart benefits. Lycopene has been linked to reducing inflammation and improving blood vessel function. Incorporate tomatoes into your diet through salads, sauces, or as a topping for whole-grain crackers to harness their heart-protective properties.

8. Garlic: Flavorful and Heart-Protective

Garlic has been celebrated for its cardiovascular benefits, including blood pressure reduction and improved cholesterol levels. Allicin, a compound found in garlic, is believed to contribute to these effects. Include garlic in your cooking to add flavor while supporting heart health.

9. Olive Oil: Mediterranean Elixir

Extra virgin olive oil is a staple in the heart-healthy Mediterranean diet. It is rich in monounsaturated fats and antioxidants, offering anti-inflammatory and heart-protective properties. Use olive oil for cooking, salad dressings, and drizzling over vegetables to enhance both taste and heart benefits.

10. Beans and Legumes: Fiber and Plant-Based Proteins

Beans, lentils, and chickpeas are excellent sources of fiber and plant-based proteins. These nutrients contribute to satiety, weight management, and overall cardiovascular health. Incorporate beans into soups, stews, or salads for a heart-healthy boost.

11. Green Tea: Antioxidant-Rich Elixir

Green tea is not only a soothing beverage but also a source of powerful antioxidants, including catechins. These compounds have been associated with improved heart health, including lower blood pressure and cholesterol levels. Swap sugary beverages for green tea to enhance your heart-protective beverage choices.

12. Red Wine: Resveratrol Benefits in Moderation

Red wine, consumed in moderation, has been linked to cardiovascular benefits due to the presence of resveratrol. This antioxidant is found in grape skins and may contribute to improved heart health. However, moderation is key, as excessive alcohol consumption can have adverse effects.

Incorporating these heart-boosting superfoods into your diet doesn't have to be daunting. Small, consistent changes can lead to significant improvements in cardiovascular health over time. Experiment with different recipes, create colorful and diverse meals, and enjoy the journey towards

a   heart-healthy   lifestyle.   Remember,   a

well-rounded and delicious diet is a key ingredient

in the recipe for a strong and resilient heart.

Chapter 13: Meal Prep and Planning for Heart Health

In the fast-paced rhythm of modern life, carving out time for wholesome, heart-healthy meals can seem like a daunting task. However, the art of meal prep and planning is a game-changer when it comes to nourishing your cardiovascular system. In this, we'll explore the significance of preparing meals in advance and how it can contribute to a proactive approach in preventing heart disease.

Understanding the Importance of Meal Prep

Meal prep involves preparing and cooking meals in advance, typically for the week ahead. This practice not only saves time but also promotes healthier eating habits. When it comes to heart health, having pre-planned meals allows you to focus on incorporating essential nutrients while avoiding impulsive, less nutritious choices.

One of the key benefits of meal prep is portion control. Overeating, especially high-calorie and high-fat foods, can contribute to weight gain and increase the risk of heart-related issues. By portioning out meals in advance, you gain better control over your calorie intake and can ensure a well-balanced diet.

Building a Heart-Healthy Meal Plan

Creating a heart-healthy meal plan begins with understanding the nutritional needs specific to cardiovascular health. Incorporating a variety of fruits, vegetables, whole grains, lean proteins, and heart-healthy fats is essential. During meal prep, aim to include a colorful array of fruits and vegetables, as they are rich in antioxidants and fiber, which play a crucial role in heart health.

Lean proteins, such as fish, poultry, beans, and legumes, provide essential amino acids without the saturated fats found in red meat. Opting for whole grains over refined grains ensures a higher intake of fiber and essential nutrients, contributing to improved cholesterol levels and overall heart function.

Efficiency and Organization in Meal Prep

Successful meal prep requires organization and efficiency. Start by planning your meals for the week, considering your schedule and nutritional needs. Create a shopping list based on your meal plan to streamline grocery shopping and avoid last-minute temptations.

Investing in quality storage containers can make a significant difference in maintaining the freshness and flavor of your prepared meals. Consider labeling containers with the date to keep track of freshness and ensure you consume meals within a safe timeframe.

Batch cooking is another time-saving technique in meal prep. Prepare larger quantities of staples like grains, proteins, and vegetables that can be used in multiple dishes throughout the week. This not only saves time but also promotes variety in your meals.

Customizing Meal Prep for Busy Lifestyles

For individuals with hectic schedules, finding time for meal prep might seem challenging, but it's crucial for maintaining heart health. Look for quick and simple recipes that require minimal preparation time. Utilize time-saving kitchen gadgets, such as a slow cooker or instant pot, to simplify the cooking process.

Consider designating specific days for meal prep, creating a routine that aligns with your lifestyle. Some find success in preparing meals for the entire week on Sundays, while others prefer to split the task between two shorter sessions during the week. Find a rhythm that works for you and helps you stay consistent with your heart-healthy meal plan.

Balancing Convenience and Nutrition

In the quest for convenience, it's essential to strike a balance between quick meals and nutritional value. While convenience foods can be time-saving, many are high in sodium, unhealthy fats, and preservatives. Opt for minimally processed options or prepare your own convenience foods during meal prep.

Snacks are an integral part of daily nutrition and can contribute significantly to heart health. Prepare heart-healthy snacks like cut fruits, vegetable sticks with hummus, or a handful of nuts during your meal prep sessions. Having nutritious snacks readily available can prevent reaching for less healthy alternatives in moments of hunger.

Meal Prep for Special Dietary Needs

Individuals with specific dietary needs, such as those following a vegetarian or gluten-free diet, can also benefit from meal prep. Planning meals in advance ensures that dietary requirements are met without compromising on taste or variety. Explore diverse recipes that align with your dietary preferences and prepare them in batches for convenience.

Educating and Involving the Whole Family

Meal prep becomes even more effective when it involves the whole family. Educate family members about the importance of heart-healthy eating and encourage their participation in meal planning and preparation. This not only shares the workload but also fosters a supportive environment for maintaining a heart-healthy lifestyle.

✒ About the Author

Lucia Diaz Mateo is a renowned cardiologist, passionate about empowering individuals to take charge of their heart health through lifestyle modifications. With over two decades of clinical experience, Lucia Diaz Mateo has dedicated her career to the prevention and treatment of cardiovascular issues.

A graduate of the prestigious Heart Institute, Lucia Diaz Mateo combines her extensive medical expertise with a deep commitment to educating the public on heart-healthy living. Her research has been published in leading medical journals, and she frequently serves as a keynote speaker at international conferences, sharing her insights on the intersection of nutrition, lifestyle, and cardiovascular wellness.

Beyond her clinical work, Lucia Diaz Mateo is a firm believer in the transformative power of accessible health information. Her writing seamlessly blends medical knowledge with practical advice, making complex concepts digestible for readers seeking to prioritize heart health.

As an advocate for holistic well-being, Lucia Diaz Mateo embodies a compassionate approach to healthcare, encouraging readers to embark on a journey of self-discovery and embrace the profound connection between their dietary choices and heart vitality.